RADICAL SELF CARE

How to Use Self Care to Thrive During Challenging Times

By

Lianne Weaver

The information in this book is not intended to replace
the advice of a physician or other medical professional.
You should consult a medical professional in matters
relating to health, especially if you have existing medical
conditions, and before starting, stopping, or changing the
dose of any medication you are taking. Individual
readers are solely responsible for their own health-care
decisions. The author and the publisher do not accept
responsibility for any adverse effects individuals may
claim to experience, whether directly or indirectly, from
the information contained in this book.

To my brilliant dad,

My supporter,

My hero,

My advisor,

My protector,

My friend,

My heart.

Always missed and forever loved.

Table of Contents

How to Get the Most from This Book

All of our Beam Series Books are designed to give you the reader the most practical tools, techniques and tips possible. The intention is never that you immediately put every single one into use but that you are inspired to start making small, sustainable changes which lead to a happier and healthier you.

As a trainer, I write with the hope that you will get the most out of this book and so would love to share some of my favourite tips to help you do that. Before we get into content, let's cover some of the basics to help you get the most out of this book.

1. **Take notes** – Really! This book has the power to change your life, but you will need to make the changes suggested in order to do so. Very few of us can recall everything we read once and if all you do is read this book once, the chances are you will forget a lot of it within a few days. When you make notes, you are ensuring your brain is more actively

involved in the learning process and so you are far more likely to retain what we cover. To supercharge this, don't make digital notes but turn to good old fashioned pen and paper!

2. **Pause** – As a fairly short book the temptation may be to consume it all in one sitting, but there will be exercises and opportunities for reflection so take an opportunity to pause and digest what is covered.

3. **There's no magic pill** – Everyone is different, our mental and emotional experiences are different, how we learn is different and our beliefs are different. That means that, unfortunately, I cannot give a one size fits all approach to any wellbeing, mental health or personal development topic. However, what I can do is offer a wide variety of tools and techniques with the intention that at least one of them will work for you.

4. **One sit up doesn't create a six pack** – On the topic of magic pills, doing these exercises once will unfortunately not yield permanent results just as one sit up does not make a six pack (darn it!). You may not notice changes initially but have faith that you are teaching your brain to respond in a different way and

eventually committing to those changes will yield positive results.

5. **All experiences are different** – Self Don't compare yourself to others and don't worry that you may have different experiences to them. If you are at all concerned about your mental or physical health, please seek help from a health professional or refer to the support services listed in this book.

6. **Don't procrastinate** – So often, we flick through a book and buy it with optimism of learning the secrets to life and then we leave it on a bookshelf (or on our ebook reader) for years and years. As much as I believe the tools in this book are powerful, not one of them is powerful enough to work if you do not even read it! Procrastination is something many of us do quite well (when the world is scary, it often feels safer to do nothing) so do not let it prevent you from making these positive changes.

7. **Use the Resources** – Within this book you will find some exercises. If you would rather complete them as worksheets, we have a range of resources available for you to download. All you need to do is scan the QR code at the end of the book or visit

https://www.beamtraining.co.uk/beamre sources and you will be able to access them.

This book is focussed upon clear ways in which we can practise practical self care to help us in all areas of our life, so please start practising self care right now by giving yourself an opportunity to sit and read in peace and quiet for at least five minutes.

Introduction

At some point in our lives, most of us have said that we wish we could have a nice, simple life, but in reality, none of us would be content with that. If we had a completely simple life with no challenges, it would become dull and flat very quickly. We would crave excitement and seek out challenges. Tony Robbins talks about how human beings have 6 core needs that we may prioritise differently, but we need all six to feel fulfilled (Certainty, Uncertainty, Significance, Connection, Growth and Contribution). All of these are interesting but the two that fascinate me are the paradoxical 'certainty and uncertainty'.

No wonder we are never satisfied. We all crave the certainty that the things we love in our life will never change and yet we all balance that with the risk of being bored and the need for the uncomfortable things in our lives to change as soon as possible. It is a knife's edge that we all walk, very rarely hitting that sweet spot with the right amount of certainty and uncertainty.

If we were to experience that simple life with no challenges, our need for uncertainty would be a powerful urge. The reality is, we need those challenges in life. We have grown far more from our challenges than we have from our good times. Think back, that difficult job, relationship, health challenge has undoubtedly changed you profoundly, but we do not always see this until we have the benefit of hindsight.

In fact, I would be as bold as to say that without those challenging times, you would also never be able to fully appreciate when life is going right.

Of course, that does not mean that we all run to the challenges thinking how much they will shape and define us in the positive. Most of us still fear them and do everything we can to avoid them.

Since 2020, we have all undergone more challenges than ever before. On a global scale we have all faced a pandemic, something we had no experience of and something which has changed our lives for ever. We have faced the threat of wars, energy crisis, cost of living crisis, politicians acting irresponsibly, public health crisis and more. In fact, you could say that, for many of us, we have encountered more global challenges in the last few years than we had in the previous few decades.

On their own, they would have all been a lot to handle, but you may have noticed that life does not give you one challenge, let you deal with that, recover and then hand you another one. No, life seems to give us multiple challenges all at the same time which can leave us feeling broken, overwhelmed, anxious, afraid, depressed, frustrated and many more difficult emotions. It is safe to assume that whilst we have been dealing with all of those global crises you have also been dealing with your own personal challenges at the same time, ranging from bereavements to financial problems to work problems and so on.

It is when we feel that we are being bombarded with challenges that we are likely to hear ourselves say "I just want a nice simple life".

Having worked in wellbeing for over a decade, I have encountered thousands of people dealing with their own challenges and one thing I know for sure is that we cannot escape them. I often describe to my clients that life is like one great big water wheel. Sometimes we are stood atop of it taking in the view, nice and dry and feeling great. We could be there for months, weeks or minutes, but eventually that wheel will continue to turn leaving us sometimes scrambling in the water whilst we pray that it will turn again and soon be over. The wheel always continues to turn - we just never know at what speed. So when we are on top we should enjoy it and take in the view, but when we are at the bottom we should find comfort in knowing that it will inevitably turn once more.

From a personal perspective, I have had more than my fair share of challenges. My life has been filled with a whole range of challenges which have often occurred simultaneously: a toxic relationship, financial loss, miscarriage, multiple bereavements, health challenges and so much more.

Over the years, I have worked hard to help pull myself out of the depths and come out of those situations stronger than when I went in. This has not always worked and has never been easy. These life experiences led me to an entire career change from accountancy into wellbeing and personal development, a career I absolutely adore but one that I originally went into for my own self-healing.

During my career, I have come to notice the cycles within our lives and have worked hard to help myself and others come out of them stronger. One of the principal ways in which I have achieved this is with my method of going back to basics and practising fundamental self care, which is entirely what this book is about. So, if you feel completely overwhelmed right now, read on and I will show you how to turn that wheel once more.

Part I: Understanding Self Care

Chapter One: The Self Care Basics

When life starts giving us challenges our stress levels rise, making it hard to focus upon anything else that is happening, we find that we are overwhelmed with the problems in front of us and therefore have neither time nor energy to deal with anything else. This is precisely when we start to neglect the self care basics.

The moment you catch yourself saying "I haven't got time to eat better" or "I don't have the energy to exercise" or "I try to sleep but it's impossible with everything I have going on!" is the moment you have lost control.

Over the last few years, I have been increasingly asked to attend events and workshops to speak on the subject of self care. It has become one of those 'buzz phrases' that you hear thrown around. It is something people feel that they should be doing but in reality do not have much of an idea what it looks like.

Many people turn to social media to get answers, which often shows self care as long bubble baths with candles, a relaxing massage or walks along the beach.

Now I would never knock a bath, massage or walk but self care is so much more than that and this is where I think we go wrong. We look for the luxurious when in reality self care is basic, fundamental and not very Instagram glamorous.

As soon as life starts spiralling out of control, it is the basics of self care that get bypassed. We then struggle to deal with our stressors whilst causing further stress on our body, mind and spirit by ignoring its core needs. This is what this book aims to address, to encourage you to care for the basics so that you have the energy and motivation to take a candlelit bubble bath now and again!

As we go through the process, we will recognise that fundamental self care is something that needs to be a consideration for all of us no matter where our mental or physical health sits.

The great aspect of this is that this relates to everyone. All of us have basic self care needs that are universal in every human being so it really does not matter who you are, what demands are placed upon you or what your stressors currently are. This book will help you care for yourself in a way that supports those inevitable life challenges.

The self care basics we will look at are:

- Sleep – How well do you sleep? Do you wake feeling rested?
- Nutrition – Are you eating food that nourishes you? Do you have good gut health?
- Movement – Are you moving enough? Are you too sedentary during the day?
- Breath – Are you breathing functionally? Do you have respiratory issues?
- Hydration – Do you drink enough water? Do you suffer with brain fog?
- Stillness – Are you able to just 'be'? Do you have moments of stillness during the day?
- Purpose – Do you have a sense of purpose? Do you feel you are making an impact in your world?

- Relationships – Do you have strong, nourishing relationships? Do you feel loved and supported?

These eight factors impact every area of our lives and when we neglect them, we quickly notice the impact it can have on us.

Before getting into the book in more detail, and learning much more about each of these aspects, it is useful to take a snapshot of where you are right now in terms of these eight basics. Fill in the Self Care Wheel which you can either see below or download from https://www.beamtraining.co.uk/beamresources.

Take some time, scoring each area out of ten, ten being 'this part of my life is amazing and could not possibly improve', one being 'this is awful and I am barely functioning here'.

There is no judgement, and you need not share this with anyone else, so be honest as it will give you a good foundation for the rest of the book and, much more importantly, for the rest of your life too.

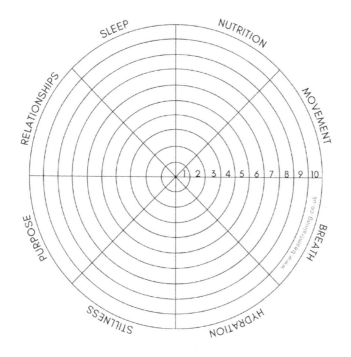

Having completed this, try not to criticise or berate yourself. The whole reason you have been drawn to this book is because you know you have areas in your life that need improving, so see this as the first step to you getting clarity and making those changes.

Key Takeaways

- When we begin to feel stressed or under pressure, we start to neglect our most basic self care.

- When thinking about self care, we can often look for the luxurious, when it is the basic acts of self care which will have the greatest impact upon us.

- Fundamental self care is an essential aspect of positive wellbeing.

- During this book we will look at self care in terms of the eight key factors of fundamental self care.

In the next chapter, you will learn...

Why we struggle with practising self care by looking at some of the barriers which prevent us from doing so.

Chapter Two: Barriers to Self Care

Having an idea of the areas within our life that we have been neglecting is useful, but you may already be asking yourself "Why do I do this to myself?" or "Why don't I make time for myself?"

You are certainly not alone. I encounter people every single day who are going through difficulties and, without having to point it out, they will acknowledge that they "should" be eating better or exercising more. Deep down, we know that what we are doing is not good for us and yet when we are struggling we cannot seem to stop ourselves from sabotaging and neglecting ourselves.

Research shows that there are many reasons for us neglecting our self care. According to The International Centre for Self Care Research, we struggle to perform self care largely due to a challenge in changing our behaviours which we hope to address within this book. Some of the most common reasons for us struggling to practice self care are:

Our Early Experiences

Our behaviours are the product of our experiences throughout our life and many are shaped from a young age. If we have unhealthy eating or exercise habits, this is often learned early on in life and therefore can be hard to change (Miller et al, 2018).

Human beings rarely learn from being told what to do. We are mimics and learn by copying the behaviour of those around us. Therefore, even if our parents told us to be kinder to ourselves, if we witnessed them being self sacrificing, people pleasing and putting their needs at the bottom of the pile, then it is highly likely we will have learned to copy that behaviour from a young age and this can seem difficult to break.

Environmental Factors

Our environment has a huge impact upon our identity. If we find ourselves in an unhealthy environment then making healthy choices can feel far more difficult. This can range from practicalities such as a lack of open or safe spaces to exercise in or even an unhealthy living environment, such as renting a crowded house share where cooking facilities are difficult to navigate.

Habit Challenges

Our habits make up much of our daily behaviour and are operated within the subconscious mind. This makes it increasingly difficult for our conscious mind to either start or stop a habit as they are often conducted when we are on 'autopilot'.

Many of our fundamental behaviours we will be tackling are habitual, such as sleep, nutrition and movement, and changing them can feel almost impossible when we are already in an established habit with them.

However, whilst it can be challenging to change a habit, it is something we have all done in our lives and we will look at the end of the book into how we can change our behaviours permanently.

Chronic Illness

Self care is seemingly never more important than when we are struggling with a chronic illness, a time when caring for ourselves and prioritising our needs would be much needed. However, this is also a time when we have little to no energy to create new habits and behaviours.

When dealing with a chronic illness much of the time, there is a need to assume responsibility and management of our own health. Out of 525,600 minutes in a year, patients with chronic conditions spend only on average 66 minutes (0.01%) of the time with a healthcare professional (Riegel et al, 2017) highlighting the need to take responsibility and invest time in managing the condition daily.

However, this is often frightening, overwhelming and daunting, leaving those with chronic conditions feeling confused, isolated and frustrated.

Selfishness

Taking time to care for our own needs often leads us to incorrectly label that as a selfish act. This mindset can come from many experiences, but it is fundamentally from our childhood when we are encouraged to compromise and collaborate with others.

As a new born baby, we are entirely self-focussed (or selfish!). We do not care that our caregiver is sleeping or eating when we want our needs met - we scream and cry until it is taken care of. This ensures our survival and is essential to our development. However, as we begin to get older, we learn that we also need to interact with a community and its survival is dependent on cooperation between each other. We are encouraged to share, to be patient with others and to understand that sometimes their needs have to get met over our own. We are rewarded for doing this and often punished with the chastisement of "Don't be so selfish" when we do not do it.

For some, this means that they can learn that the needs of others are more important than their own needs, causing them to learn to always self sacrifice and put their own needs at the bottom of the list. For these people, being called selfish would be a huge insult and cause emotional pain, embarrassment and, for some, even shame.

Guilt

Tying into selfishness is the heavy burden of guilt we may feel if or when we do anything that is entirely for ourselves. We believe that doing something for ourselves is 'wrong' in some way and start to feel guilty.

As an emotion, guilt only carries a moment of worth, beyond which it is useless. This worth is to inspire us to take corrective action when our behaviour has not matched up to our own moral code. For example, you realise that yesterday was your friend's birthday and you had completely forgotten about it. You feel that pang of guilt which encourages you to take corrective action by sending a belated card or gift, making a phone call and apologising. The guilt has been helpful.

However, many of us feel guilt for things we either do not take corrective action over or we have no corrective action to take. In the case of self care, this often means we feel guilty because we spent a whole hour to ourselves and did not clean the house. We cannot go back in time and clean the house in that hour, it has passed. This leaves us feeling persistently guilty and as though we should have done better.

If you are not sure if guilt is holding you back, a sure fire way to identify if guilt is playing a role in your life is to pay attention to the language you use. If you use the word 'should' a lot, especially when talking to yourself, then you are sure to be struggling with guilt.

"Should", in my opinion, is the most toxic word we use. It makes us feel unworthy, guilty and resentful. Imagine your friend calls to your house and after half an hour of chatting they say "you should make me a cup of tea". You are likely to have one of two reactions, or a mix of both, where you either feel guilty for being a bad host and a little embarrassed and ashamed or you feel annoyed by their request which causes you to feel resentment. This is the impact of 'should-ing' yourself - a mixture of guilt and resentment causing you to feel not good enough.

Busy-ness

As a society, we have slipped into measuring our worth and value by how busy we are. Some people wear their busy-ness as a badge of honour, making claims like "I haven't had time to eat today" or "I don't get to sit down until around midnight".

I have heard almost every excuse for why someone is too busy to look after themselves and unfortunately, not one of them holds up.

Being relentlessly busy is not a badge of honour but something which will negatively impact almost every area of your life. As the phrase goes, "We are human beings, not human doings" and it is essential for us to slow down and learn to just be rather than continually feeling like we have to produce.

People Pleasing

Are you a people pleaser? Do you always worry what other people will think or say if you do not go along with them? People pleasing is something I used to believe was more of a personality trait than anything else, but it is not. People pleasing is a response we learn to engage in whenever we feel stressed in order for us to appease the stressor.

The problem with constantly people pleasing is that we rarely end up pleasing ourselves. In fact, every single time we say yes to doing something we do not want to do for someone else, we are saying a no to ourselves.

As a people pleaser, you are likely to neglect your own needs because you consistently overvalue everyone else above yourself. In fact you will find that your name is usually at the very bottom of your to do list.

When we people please, we create a rule that everybody's needs are more important than our own. But this is simply not true; our needs are just as important as everyone else's.

More often than not, we forget to prioritise our self care due to a combination of all of these reasons (and some extra ones too which we may have learned through our relationships with others). It is important for us to realise that these reasons are not rules that we must adhere to. In fact we need to recognise that practising some fundamental self care will not only benefit us, but those around us too.

Throughout this book we will be mindful of these challenges and begin to make positive changes in small but meaningful ways in order for us to reap the rewards.

Exercise

Spend some time reflecting on the below questions to identify some of your barriers to self care now. If you would prefer, these questions are also available in a printable worksheet from our website resources.

Q1.　If I had an unexpected day to myself, what would I do?

Q2.　Do I feel guilty if I put my needs first?

Q3.　How would I feel if someone called me selfish?

Q4.　When was the last time I did something just for myself?

Key Takeaways

- Even though we may be aware that we need to care for ourselves more, there are common barriers that prevent us and cause us to self sabotage our best intentions.

- Some reasons for a lack of self care are:

  a. We have learned some poor behaviours from childhood which feel hard to overcome and change.

b. We may find ourselves in an environment which does not support the healthier changes we would like to make.

c. We struggle with chronic illness and lack energy, direction or motivation to know how to make positive changes.

d. We believe others may see it as selfish or we consider it to be selfish.

e. We feel guilty doing things for ourselves.

f. We are constantly busy, causing us to believe that we do not have the time nor energy to do things for ourselves.

g. We feel we should people please, prioritising the needs of others over our own.

In the next chapter, you will learn...

Why practising self care is so beneficial to our overall wellbeing.

Chapter Three: The Benefits of Self Care

Despite there being challenges which act as barriers to us practising self care, when we begin to make a commitment to care for ourselves we can start to see many benefits to our health, happiness, relationships and more.

There are thousands of research papers on self care (it is difficult to put an exact number on it as there are multiple terms and synonyms used for self care) with the first being published in 1946. These research studies show time and time again that self care has huge benefits on our mental, physical and spiritual wellbeing.

When we practise self care regularly it is frequently shown that we become more resilient, handle stress better, feel happier and even live longer.

It Makes us More Resilient

True resilience is about being resourceful enough to face a challenging situation. Self care and self compassion are some of the key resources we need in order to face challenges and bounce back from adversity.

As we have already learned, when we face a challenge in our lives one of the first things that often gets neglected is our own basic needs. When we become better at making sure our most basic of needs are benefitting us, then we are likely to feel mentally and physically stronger in any situation. Furthermore, the practice of paying attention to our own needs can often ensure that we do not reach burnout and recognise warning signs earlier on that we are in need of some support or a break.

It Makes us Prioritise Ourselves

One of the biggest sources of discontent I see in the therapy room is the feeling of overwhelm and as though we no longer matter. I cannot count the number of clients I have sat opposite who have told me how they wish the people around them recognised that they were struggling and needed help.

Many of us can find ourselves in a situation where we hope that others will see that we are struggling and almost await their 'permission' for us to rest or take care of ourselves. You do not need anybody's permission to take care of yourself, you just need to take the first step.

When we value ourselves in this way, we are less likely to be running on empty and more likely to be able to enforce boundaries that protect us from total exhaustion; in summary it helps us prioritise ourselves.

It Improves Self Awareness

Being self aware is knowing and understanding yourself, being able to understand why you behave in a certain way, why you respond in a certain way and knowing what matters to you and why. Self awareness is the foundation stone of developing emotional intelligence, having the ability to understand yourself and others.

When we continually sacrifice our own needs to benefit and serve others, we start to disconnect from who we are and what we need. We silence the nagging internal voice that whispers "I need to rest" or "I can't do this" and keep pushing onwards.

When we prioritise our basic needs we develop a relationship with ourselves that extends beyond having to do things and moves us towards being self compassionate and self nurturing. You will be more likely to know times that you may be oversensitive, overreact or overwhelmed and will develop the awareness to notice your patterns of behaviour and understand what you may need to help avoid feeling that way.

It Helps us Set Boundaries

As you begin to recognise your own needs, you may notice that you start to become protective of your exercise time, you meal time, your sleep or nurturing the relationships which are good for you. When we start to develop this level of self awareness we can become better at setting boundaries with others, preventing us from feeling used and overwhelmed.

Boundaries are how we communicate to others what is and is not okay. We tend to assume that others will be able to recognise our boundaries without ever communicating them and then become insulted when people overstep them.

Boundaries need to be communicated and the more you can recognise your own needs, the easier that will be. Here are some examples:

I don't look at my emails after 6pm.

I don't take my phone to bed.

I always go for a walk at 8am.

I always take a lunch break.

Setting clear boundaries are an important part of self care and will help you to regain control of your time and energy.

Key Takeaways

- Practising self care can help us to be more resilient and to recognise when we need extra support.

- When we begin to practise self care, we no longer need to wait for permission from others to take care of our needs.

- Acts of self care help us get to know ourselves better and improve our self awareness.

- When we begin to see the benefits of self care, it becomes easier to set clear boundaries with others.

In the next chapter, you will learn...

About the self care basics, as we begin to explore all eight of the key areas of self care and look at ways in which you can improve your scores in them. We will begin by looking at sleep.

Part II: The Self Care Basics

Chapter Four: Sleep

Sleep occupies around a third of our life. The National Sleep Foundation suggests that we need 7-9 hours of sleep a night and yet most of us give our sleep health very little attention until it becomes an issue in our lives.

When we sleep well we rarely consider it and yet as soon as we suffer one sleepless night we become acutely aware of the impact a lack of sleep can have upon our mental and physical health.

You may be one of those people who states that they only have 5 hours sleep a night and can operate totally fine on it. However, science disagrees with you. Neuroscientist and Sleep Expert, Matthew Walker, has stated that from his research, it is clear that anyone who is getting less than 6 hours sleep a night is not thriving and very few of us can routinely operate on such little sleep (so few, according to Walker, that if it was rounded to a whole number it would equate to 0%).

We certainly know from our own personal experience that when we lose even one night of sleep we are impacted heavily, we may struggle to concentrate, suffer from low or poor mood, have poorer decision making ability, have slower reaction times and be more likely to feel unwell.

Sleep is not only crucial for our mental wellbeing, but it is also an essential aspect of repairing, cleansing and renewing our cells and organ functions. Every single aspect of our physical and mental health is in fact impacted by sleep. When we get enough we are more resilient, when we do not get enough we are weaker.

Why Can't I Sleep?

Sleep is such a crucial part of our wellbeing that it seems paradoxical that during the times we need sleep the most – when under pressure – we struggle to achieve it. Of course, having a period of sleeplessness is perfectly normal and is something we will all experience, which is often due to stress and / or illness, but most of us then revert back to our normal healthy sleeping pattern once this has passed.

However, for some of us, sleep can be forever elusive and something we seem to struggle with frequently. It is incredibly important here to note that lacking sleep, whilst normal from time to time, can be an indicator of underlying health issues so prolonged and / or unexplained lack of sleep is something you should always discuss with a health professional.

Here are a few of the principal reasons many of us struggle with our sleep:

- **We don't value it** – According to sleep experts this is the top reason that we struggle with sleep. We tend to see sleep as a passive activity which should just happen to us, but we actually need to invest some time and energy into creating a healthy sleep pattern. If we see sleep as an inconvenience, something we do not really have time for, or something which is a waste of time, we prevent ourselves from seeing the value in it.

- **Inconsistency** – Every sleep expert I have ever listened to mentions one key requirement for healthy sleep, which is regularity. Many of us have an inconsistent sleep schedule, waking early on weekdays, laying in on weekends or having to work alternate shift patterns. This prevents the brain from creating a pattern for sleep and causes us to have many wakeful moments.

- **Screen Use** – Our exposure to screens has a huge impact upon our ability to sleep. A study in 2021, (Wagner et al, 2021) found that Americans in their mid-twenties spent on average 28.5 hours per week staring at screens. Not only does this connect to eye strain, obesity and mental health issues, but it significantly connects to poor sleep. Staring at screens has been shown to impair our brains' ability to trigger the production of melatonin (a hormone essential for helping us fall to sleep) and exposing ourselves to information which potentially causes us stress before sleep leads to an increase in the stress hormone cortisol, which impedes our ability to fall asleep.

- **Anxiety** – When we feel anxious, we are likely to overthink and have higher levels of stress hormones in our system, especially cortisol. Cortisol is produced to protect us from an imminent threat and as it rises, it has a huge impact upon our neurochemistry and physiology. One being, that as cortisol increases, melatonin (the hormone needed to help us fall to sleep) decreases.

- **Caffeine** – We all know that caffeine is a stimulant and is something that keeps us awake but we may not realise that caffeine has a half life of around 5 to 6 hours. This means that if you drink a cup of coffee at 6pm, it will still be in your system at 12am. Caffeine not only stimulates us to make us feel more awake, but it also masks our fatigue and so a late night cup of coffee may mean we do not even realise we are tired.

- **Alcohol** – Many people will think that having an alcoholic drink helps them go off to sleep but alcohol is highly disruptive to our sleep. This means that both the quality and quantity of sleep we get after a few drinks is impaired.

- **Tobacco** – You may be less aware that smoking is also a stimulant and, in the same way as caffeine, masks your fatigue causing your brain to not realise that you are indeed tired.

- **Eating too late** – This is something we will cover in more detail when we come to the nutrition part of the book. When we eat late at night, our body needs to use its energy to digest the meal at a time when it should be slowing down and help us rest for repair and renewal. Guidelines vary but in my experience, stopping eating a minimum of three hours before sleep has a huge positive impact on both quantity and quality of sleep.

- **Exercising too late** – Exercise is brilliant for sleep but it appears that it is most beneficial when done earlier in the day. If we exercise too near to our bed time we can not only be overstimulated but crucially, we increase our core body temperature, which needs to be lowered in order for us to have restful sleep.

- **Our environment** – The place you sleep is very important to your quality of sleep. Is your bedroom a relaxing environment? If it is full of clutter, if you have lots of screens and technology in it, if it is too light or if it is too warm, your sleep is likely to be negatively affected.

How to Improve Sleep

When we struggle with sleep it is first wise to ensure that there are no health reasons for this. Insomnia is defined as having difficulty maintaining or initiating sleep for a period of at least three times per week for more than one month. If this sounds like you then again I suggest a conversation with your GP to rule out any health issues.

However, if there are no obvious health issues then there are things we can do to help us get back into a healthy pattern of sleeping once more.

Before we look at those tools, it is important to say something here that may sound difficult to practise but if you are lacking sleep, try not to worry and overfocus upon it. Many people can become fixated on thinking "I must have 8 hours of sleep" and that in itself becomes enough to disrupt the sleeping pattern. At this stage, I would avoid those thoughts and settle more on "I am improving my sleep hygiene" which will help you maintain focus but will avoid counterproductive goal setting.

41

Prioritise Your Sleep

In terms of our mental and physical health, there are few things that can have such a drastic impact in such a short space of time than sleep. Since the Industrial Revolution, sleep has been seen as something that is of less and less importance and almost as an inconvenience to our lives. This is not only unhelpful but is also untrue.

When we begin to value sleep, we make space for it in our lives as an important part of our self care routine. Without it, many of the other tools we will learn in this book will become harder and harder to practise.

The first step to better sleep is therefore making a commitment to see it as an essential part of your wellbeing and something that, from today, you will prioritise.

What's Your Sleep Story?

Sleep Physiologist, Dr Guy Meadows, who helps insomniacs improve their sleep, talks about our 'sleep story' and how powerful that can be for our overall relationship with sleep.

Consider your own sleep story. Do you say things like "I always wake at 3am" or "I never get off to sleep easily" or "I can't sleep without a drink" or "I always need to go to the loo at least twice a night". Whilst these stories may seem entirely factual right now, they are powerful enough to keep you trapped in a cycle of poor sleep.

When someone is a good sleeper, they do not talk about it very much. If questioned they are likely to simply say "I sleep well". Their sleep story is simple and something which will not prevent them from a good sleep habit.

If you have realised you have a negative sleep story, start by making that simpler and more positive, even if it does not feel true in this moment. Here are some simple but effective sleep stories you could start saying whenever you think about sleep:

- I sleep well.

- I always get enough sleep.

- I enjoy sleeping.

- I always wake up revitalised.

Again, notice that these sleep stories are not intended to create pressure and anxiety over sleep, so avoid making statements such as "I always get at least 8 hours of sleep" or "I never need to wake up for a bathroom break".

Be Consistent

Every sleep expert I have ever listened to has always given this one piece of advice … Be consistent!

The worst sleepers amongst us have poor sleep routines. They may go to bed at a wide variety of times or have long lie-ins on the weekend. Whilst this is difficult for those of you who work shifts, if you are able to be consistent with your bed and waking times, your brain will settle into that pattern far more easily than if it fluctuates.

Although it can be tempting to stay up late and laze in bed on the weekend, avoid doing so if you want to create a healthy sleep pattern. Your circadian rhythm does not realise (or care) what day of the week it is and so upsetting your sleep cycle will upset the circadian rhythm.

Create Darkness

Before electricity we were largely wired to sleep when it got dark and wake when it became light. This of course changed with the introduction of household electricity when we could create artificial light which would trick the brain into staying awake longer.

In order for the sleep hormone, melatonin, to be produced, we need to begin to create darkness. Avoiding LED lights, bright lamps and of course screens will all help prepare the brain for sleep.

Consider having blackout curtains or blinds in your bedroom and even an eye mask to help create that darkness no matter what time of day it is you need to sleep (especially important if you work shifts and need to sleep in the day).

Create a Sleep Routine

When we care for a new baby / young child, we tend to be very focussed upon their sleep routines. We know that sleep is essential for their growth, development and their ability to thrive and so we encourage it as much as we can by creating strong sleep routines for the child. This can include a warm drink, soft lights, a bed time story, speaking softly, avoiding anything over stimulating and going to bed at the same time every night.

Many new parents can become obsessed with their baby's sleep routine and with good reason. They know that when the baby has been prepared for sleep well, they are likely to sleep longer and wake up full of energy.

Despite us recognising this in young children, as we get older much of this tends to go out of the window. We forget about the routines and the regularity and start to create overstimulation for the entire day, which impacts our ability to sleep. Into adulthood this can become so bad that we fall into bed mentally exhausted but are incapable of sleeping for hours as our brain is too stimulated. We have simply forgotten to create a healthy sleep routine for ourselves.

Sleep routines can vary and it is important to do what works for you and what will fit into your lifestyle best. The key once again is consistency and regularity. The brain is highly associative, so if you do the same thing every night just before you sleep (and only before you sleep) your brain will soon recognise it as a trigger for sleep.

Here is an example of things to consider when creating your own sleep routine:

- Start 60 - 90 mins before – Melatonin is a slow release hormone which needs to build up in our system in order for us to feel sleepy. It is therefore useful to start a sleep routine at least an hour before you want to sleep.

- Avoid blue screens – As we have already learned, exposure to bluescreens is repeatedly shown to impair our ability to sleep. Phones and tablets are most likely to disrupt our sleep due to how close we hold them and how engrossed we can become in them, but even watching the TV will have a negative impact.

- Turn down lights – Remember that the brain needs to recognise darkness to sleep so it is important to create a quiet and dark environment wherever possible. Consider using lamps and lower lights after 9pm.

- Choose a relaxing activity – With young children we tend to give them a warm bath and / or read a story. This association creates the expectation of sleep. Consider a relaxing activity you can do every evening to create the same association, for example reading a book, doing some yoga, doing a breathing exercise.

• Expect sleep – Remember your own sleep story and if you notice a negative sleep story sneaking in, silently repeat to yourself your new positive sleep story.

Key Takeaways

• Sleep is crucial for every aspect of our physical and mental wellbeing.

• A recurring lack of sleep can be a sign of an underlying health issue and should be investigated.

• Periods of sleeplessness are normal and are usually caused by stress and / or illness.

• There are many reasons we struggle to sleep.

• Our sleep can be improved in a number of ways once we begin to prioritise it.

- Creating a sleep routine will help create an expectation of sleep.

In the next chapter, you will learn...

How movement is an essential part of our mental and physical health and how it can benefit us especially when we are dealing with a challenge.

Chapter Five: Movement

When we think of self care and wellbeing, many of us will think about the importance of exercise. If you are someone who enjoys exercise, you will already be aware that it not only helps you feel physically better but that there are huge mental benefits to exercising.

However, for some people even the term "exercise" has negative connotations. Not everyone has had a positive experience with exercise and it can conjure up images of running miles in agony or sweating in a gym full of people. This in itself can be enough to repel someone from even considering the importance of exercise to their mental health.

In addition to this, we also need to consider that whilst exercise has many benefits, when we talk about self care what we are always being mindful of is consistency during our every day life, not one off periods of exercise.

Therefore, when looking at self care, we talk about movement and its benefits over that of exercise.

The Difference Between Movement & Exercise

For the benefit of clarity, when we talk about movement in this book, we are not talking about exercise in the way that many of us may consider it. It will therefore help to define both words in the context of this book.

Exercise – "An activity requiring physical effort, carried out to sustain or improve health and fitness".

Movement – "An act of moving the body".

Whilst both movement and exercise certainly constitute by a part of self care and wellbeing, we are going to focus largely upon movement with a view to that leading to exercise.

The Problem with Sitting Still

As a species, human beings evolved to be active. Developmental molecular biologist, Dr John Medina, suggests that the human brain evolved by our ancestors walking around 12 miles per day. When you consider our ancestors, they had to move all day long in order to ensure they fed their tribe and kept them safe and warm.

Even if we forget our hunter gatherer ancestors and focus more on recent times, we could consider our grandparents, they still moved far more than we do – an estimated 30% more even in the 1960s!

The world in which we live now has unfortunately created a species of humans who can achieve most of their needs in an entirely sedentary fashion. No longer do we need to hunt for our food. In fact we no longer even have to go to a supermarket for our food and cook it - we can now order cuisine from an app on our phone which arrives within 30 minutes.

We now find ourselves living in a world where we consider a need (or want) and can receive instant gratification for it within minutes. We have even become so sedentary and lazy that now we argue about who will answer the door to the delivery person who brings the food!

Every aspect of our lives has changed over the last fifty years - how we eat, how we work, how we are entertained and how we interact. Whilst there may well be numerous positive impacts to these changes, a clear negative one is how lazy it is making us. Our desire for convenience and technological progress is having a detrimental effect on not only our physical wellbeing but also our mental wellbeing. Recent research suggests that today, we spend an incredible 70% of our lives sitting still. Being this sedentary, not only impacts our physical wellbeing but also our mental wellbeing.

Research is now highlighting that sitting still is one of the greatest risk factors to our overall health, with a research study from Mandasger, Harb, Cremer et al in 2018 finding that being sedentary posed a three times higher risk of death than smoking.

In fact, if we return to the research of Dr John Medina, he proposes that one of the greatest predictors of successful aging is the absence of a sedentary lifestyle.

Welcoming More Movement

When we are still, our body decides to conserve energy and one of the ways it does that is by slowing down our brains. It is only when we get moving that our mind is put back into motion. Being still therefore prevents us from using the most creative and resourceful aspects of ourselves.

Moving our body increases our blood flow and helps us to think more clearly. It is a practice that goes back thousands of years when many of the Stoics would walk to help them gather their thoughts.

"We should take wandering outdoor walks, so that the mind might be nourished and refreshed." – Seneca

However, it is not just ancient wisdom that talks of the benefits of moving in order for us to think better. Modern science also supports this philosophy.

Dr Kelly McGonigal (The Joy Of Movement) talks about there being a specific number of steps we need to take for positive mental health. When I ask people what they think this number would be, they almost always say 10,000 steps due to the publicity walking 10,000 steps a day has received. However, walking 10,000 steps has no science behind it. This figure came from a Japanese company who created one of the first pedometers and they named it "Manpo-Kei" which translates to 10,000 steps meter. This took off and soon everyone believed that they needed to walk 10,000 steps a day.

Whilst walking 10,000 steps will certainly benefit you, the research McGonigal discusses in her book The Joy of Movement may feel far more achievable for some of you. A research study found that in order to achieve positive mental health, participants needed to walk at least 5,649 steps per day. This study found that when participants achieved this, their experience of depression, anxiety and lack of purpose all reduced. Yet when participants were encouraged not to achieve this, 88% of them found that their experience of anxiety, depression and lack of purpose all increased.

Therefore, in order to improve our mental health, our ability to think more clearly and to feel as though we have more purpose, we need to be aiming for an overall daily step count of at least 5,649.

In addition to this, it is important we consider the idea of movement over exercise once again.

I have worked with many people who are physically fit. They exercise every day and have worked hard to create a strong physique. However sometimes these clients still present with overwhelm, anxiety and lack of resilience. Regularly, when probing their movement throughout the day, there is a clear lack of movement outside of their designated exercise time.

You may indeed go to the gym every morning for an hour and totally smash it there, running 5km, lifting weights and come out drenched in sweat. However, if you got up, drove to the gym, did your exercise, drove to work, sat at your desk, drove home, sat on your sofa, went to bed and repeat, you often realise that much of the 23 remaining hours of the day were entirely sedentary.

When we consider movement along with exercise we therefore help to keep our body and mind engaged, active and resilient.

Moving More

Consider your own situation right now. Are you spending much of your day sedentary? Would you hit that average of 70% of your time being sat still? If so, then this is your sign to start to bring more movement into your day. This can be done in small ways which you can fit into your existing day, but here are some suggestions:

- If you have a smart watch, adjust the settings so it reminds you to move if you have been sat still for too long.

- Aim to stand and move for at least 3 minutes within every hour.

- Consider bending your knees when moving. We have a key artery behind the knees which helps blood flow to the heart when moved.

- Bring small habits of movement into your existing habits, for example doing some squats as the kettle boils, pacing the room when you need to think, parking in a far away parking spot, taking the stairs not the lift.

Key Takeaways

- Whilst exercise is vital to positive wellbeing, it is movement which is fundamental to our mental wellbeing.

- The average person spends 70% of their day being sedentary.

- Being sedentary is a greater risk factor of death than smoking.

- Research found that walking 5,649 steps per day improves our mental health.

- Finding small ways to move more throughout the day will help combat being sedentary.

In the next chapter, you will learn...

How important good nutritional habits are when caring for ourselves.

Chapter Six: Nutrition

As with movement, this chapter is not intended to give you dietary advice. The health and wellbeing section of any bookstore is currently full of advice on what and how we should eat.

However, if we are talking about self care, it would be remiss to not consider the fuel we are putting into our bodies and so this chapter is designed to help you think about how you are fuelling yourself and the positive and / or negative impact that may be having on your overall wellbeing.

Many people report to me that when they are stressed and under pressure, their eating habits become instantly impacted, from people who feel so stressed they feel they cannot eat to people who constantly eat when they have a challenge.

Food is certainly one of the most complicated substances we have a relationship with. In my experience, every single person I have ever met has at some point abused food, whether that is being so busy and distracted you deny yourself food, to overindulging in your favourite snack or takeaway and then feeling or being sick as a result. Because of this, many people who struggle with their relationship with food find themselves in a repeating negative cycle of behaviour.

With most other substances, if we recognise something is harming us, we usually have the opportunity to abstain from it (alcohol for example). But with food we cannot abstain from it which can make it feel almost impossible to end an unhealthy cycle.

Our food of course nourishes and impacts our physical bodies but many of us are simply unaware of how much it also impacts our mental health. We simply have not connected the dots between how a food makes us feel physically and how it makes us feel mentally. Simply put, your food changes your mood.

When we talk about nutrition within self care, we are not discussing 'good' or 'bad' foods but rather noticing how you respond to foods and how you consume them. It is important to note that I do not believe that there is one 'magic' diet that works for all people at every stage in their lives. We all carry different genetic history, live in different environments, and need different amounts of vitamins and minerals at different points in our lives. Therefore, we are not talking about a diet plan rather to educate ourselves on the food we are now exposed to and importantly to learn what walks for our own individual bodies. To do this, when working with clients, we often create some key rules for nutrition which allow them to regain control and do what is right for them.

Eat Real Food

According to gut health charity Guts UK, people tend to not prioritise their gut health compared to their weight, sleep, teeth and heart health. And yet in the UK alone, 43% of the population have some sort of digestive dysfunction and we know that our gut health plays a huge role in our mental wellbeing.

Gut problems are on the increase and many gut experts will tell you that a big part of that is down to the diet we now consume compared to the diets our grandparents would have eaten.

"Eat Real Food" sounds like such a simple and obvious rule, and yet it is becoming increasingly more and more difficult for us to do this in a world that markets processed food to us from all angles.

The most simple interpretation of this is that if we eat chemicals, it not only can disrupt our highly delicate balanced internal ecosystem, but it also is very difficult for our body to process food which is unnatural.

In order to become better at eating real food, we unfortunately need to become smarter shoppers and read between the lines of what is being advertised to us. More often than not, if something is being deliberately marketed to us as healthy and good for us, we need to be suspicious!

Having true and accurate information about our food is difficult and many of us have become confused. For every healthy food you hear about, you can also find a study which tells you that the same food is harmful to you. This leads many people to feeling so confused that they give up and follow their tastebuds instead of the instincts.

So how on earth do we make sense of it all? I take a very simplistic view here with a few key rules which you can choose to follow:

1. Read the ingredients – if you wouldn't have an item in your food cupboard, do not eat it.

2. Be smart about the ingredients – foods must be labelled with their ingredients in order of their quantity in the food. For example, if you were buying strawberry jam you would expect strawberry to be first, then sugar etc. However, many manufacturers use varieties of the same category of ingredient so as to list it lower. Now we may notice the jam is labelled like this:

   Strawberry (40%), Sugar (32%), Cane Sugar (18%) etc

By listing two types of sugar, we now see that sugar is the majority ingredient rather than strawberries. It is worth noting here that according to UCSF's Sugar Science website there are at least 61 different names for sugar, so we need to be smart about reading those labels!

3. Fewer ingredients are better – keep your food shop simple. Aim for fewer ingredients per product.

4. Avoid processed food – processed food usually contains more chemicals and less nutrition so as much as possible avoid all processed food.

5. Choose quality over quantity – It is difficult when shopping on a budget not to get caught up in the meal deals and big portions but those meal deals and special offers are often not as nutritious.

Give Your Digestion A Rest

One of the most amazing parts of my own self care journey was understanding how I was overloading my digestive system. In 2019, I suffered awful food poisoning from a trip to India. This was not treated correctly and left me with gastric problems for two years becoming chronically ill. At the time, doctors were not sure what was wrong with me, and I became increasingly unwell. With little medical support (especially during The Pandemic, a time when we were unable to see the GP easily) I began to take matters into my own hands and learn about healing my digestive system and restoring my gut health.

This led to making numerous changes, but one was recognising how hard my gut (and yours!) works. Ancestrally, we would have had long periods of time where we did not eat, and we certainly did not eat three meals a day plus snacks. I realised that whilst I did not eat a lot, I was eating frequently and often would have an evening meal only an hour or so before bed.

I started to understand that my overworked and poorly digestive system needed to at least rest a little more. I figured that if I had a knee injury, there would be times when I would need to rest up and let it heal and repair and decided to apply similar logic to my gut.

Whilst I applied various intermittent fasting techniques, for me, the best system was with the most simplistic approach to begin with. To **not** eat for longer than I did eat.

I started to set an eating curfew for myself to ensure that I had a minimum of 14 hours rest with a 10 hour window of eating. I also learned that for improved sleep function, it is best to stop eating at least 3 hours before you sleep. I therefore stopped eating by 6pm and did not eat again until at least 8am.

To say this has been life changing is no exaggeration. Of course, I am only giving my experience here. But in today's society, we rarely allow ourselves to feel truly hungry and see mild hunger as a negative thing. However, when we stop overloading our digestive system, the body can work at a much more optimal level.

Of course, to begin with you may believe you are hungry by 9pm but this is more of a habit than a fact, indeed I started to see those hunger pangs as a sign that my body was being able to do the work it needs to do.

Abstaining from food for this period of time allows the body to regulate, repair and heal in a way it simply cannot do if it is constantly trying to digest the next meal or snack.

Pay Attention to How You Feel

As we have already discussed, there are thousands of conflicting pieces of data out there about every kind of food you can imagine. Today avocados are great for you, tomorrow they are harming you. This confusion stops us from paying attention to the most important guide we have - our own bodies.

Our food directly impacts our mood, energy levels and physiology yet we regularly ignore the messages a food is giving us.

The best way to know what food you should be eating is to ignore the outside noise and pay attention to how your brain and body responds to it. If you eat bread and instantly bloat, your body is struggling to process it and it is not something that is doing you good. If you eat sugar and your energy dies soon after, your body is again under more strain than necessary. Most of us are sensitive to some foods and of course, some of us have allergies. A sensitivity means that we can consume that food, but it may cause us to a minor physical reaction such as bloating, diarrhoea, nausea, gas etc. An allergy, however, is far more serious and that food substance must be avoided.

It is not just the stereotypical 'good' and 'bad' foods either. Sometimes we force ourselves to eat a food without paying attention to how it makes us feel because we have been told that it is good for us. Whilst apples or carrots or salad may be good for lots of people, it does not always mean they are good for you.

Your gut is constantly talking to you, so slow down your eating and start to pay more attention to what that food does to you.

One of my biggest lessons when healing my gut was understanding that the food I thought I loved may not have loved me back. One of my all time favourite comfort foods was always macaroni cheese. I craved it, I loved it and I ate it whenever I saw it on a menu. However, after having it one day I became unwell, I bloated, had stomach cramps and felt totally drained.

I chatted to my friend and brilliant EFT Practitioner, Sam Neffendorf, and told him about my experience with my favourite comfort food and his reply forever changed my relationship with it. He said "The problem is, you're calling it comfort food but in reality it is **dis**-comfort food!". What a lightbulb moment! Recognising that it didn't matter how much I thought I loved something, if it was causing me pain then it certainly was not loving me back!

This change of mindset meant that I immediately was able to change my relationship with macaroni cheese (and a few other foods) and whenever presented with the option of having them, to this day. I remind myself that they are **discomfort** foods.

Our relationship with food is highly emotional and complex but starting to recognise how we use food and how it makes us feel, especially when we are under pressure, can help us to take better care of our nutrition when we most need it.

Key Takeaways

- Our food changes our mood.

- Eating real food will support us getting the most nutritional value from our meals.

- Resting our digestive system can improve our mood and sleep amongst many other things.

- Our body will let us know if a food is good or bad for us, but we have learned to ignore the signs it gives us.

- Just because we enjoy a certain food does not mean our body benefits from it. Pay attention to any 'dis-comfort' foods you may be eating.

In the next chapter, you will learn...

How important it is to ensure you are fully hydrated throughout the day.

Chapter Seven: Hydration

We understand that food can affect our mood, but we need to also be aware that one of the most fundamental parts of caring for ourselves is ensuring we are properly hydrated.

Research shows that dehydration has a negative impact not only on our cognitive ability (our memory and perception for example) but also on our mood overall (Masento et al, 2014). This particular research study also found that sufficient hydration improved cognitive performance, visual attention and mood.

Yet, as with our connection to food, many of us have also started to ignore our body's signals that we need to drink water and / or confuse with a signal that we are hungry instead. We also have become poor at drinking pure water. Many people tell me that they don't like the taste and have to add flavour to their water.

Paying attention to our hydration can have a positive measurable effect on our physical and emotional health, so again we will look at three simple rules to follow.

Drink Like a Sponge

The way we drink is more important than we may think. Many of us, when we realise we are thirsty, grab a drink and down it all in one go. When we do this, we flood our system so most of that fluid goes into our bloodstream, is filtered out into the kidneys and passed into our urine very quickly. This means that, despite consuming lots of liquid, our cells and organs will not get the benefit of rehydrating from the drink.

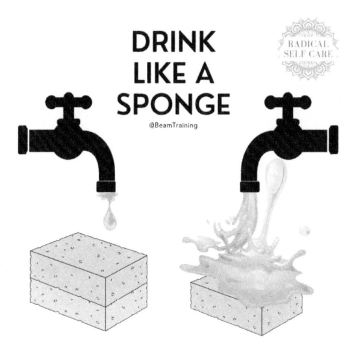

DRINK LIKE A SPONGE

@BeamTraining

A great way to think about how we hydrate is to consider how you would put water onto a sponge. If you have a sponge and place it under a tap with the tap on at full capacity, the sponge will not soak up very much of that water as it will bounce off it. However, if you place the sponge under the tap and leave the tap to slowly drip, the sponge can soak up the majority of the water. Take a look at the diagram above to see this illustrated.

According to Dr Scott Blossom (Doctor of Traditional Chinese Medicine and Ayurveda), the body can absorb about an ounce of water every 10 minutes, so if we overdrink our body will immediately start to filter the excess water and we get the urge to urinate quickly.

We know that feeling fully hydrated is essential for us to feel alert and healthy. It therefore is crucial for us to become better at how we consume our water and slow things down.

Don't Drink Your Sugar

One of the most damaging things we do to our body is drinking highly sweet drinks (whether that is with sugar or artificial sweeteners).

Dr Mark Hyman (Author of Food Fix) stated that "cutting sugar-sweetened beverages from your diet is the single biggest thing you can do to improve your health". This powerful statement highlights how damaging our addiction to sugary drinks is to our health.

This of course includes soda and energy drinks, but it also includes fruit juice. Many of us have been led to believe that drinking fruit juices is good for us. However they contain huge amounts of sugar that we know are harmful to our health. Tom Rath (Author of Eat, Move, Sleep) states "Sugar is a toxin. It fuels diabetes, obesity, heart disease and cancer."

We also know that consuming excess sugar impacts our overall mood. When our blood sugar is either too high or too low, it impacts how our brain functions causing changes to our mood.

Notice Dehydration

When we become dehydrated, there are a whole host of changes which can happen in our body and in our moods. Of course, severe dehydration is dangerous and something for which you need to seek medical attention urgently. But many of us do not recognise the symptoms of mild dehydration within ourselves as a sign that we need to increase our fluid intake.

Here are a few of the more common symptoms of mild dehydration:

- Difficulty concentrating

- Memory impairment

- Headaches

- Dizziness / Lightheaded

- Decreased urination

- Fatigue

If you unexpectedly feel any of these symptoms mildly, it may be worth sipping some water to see if that eases the situation. It is also worth prioritising a glass of water first thing in the morning before you have consumed your normal mug of coffee. In the morning, we are likely to be most dehydrated after going a long period of time without fluid, being warm in our beds and possibly snoring and dribbling! All of which lead to dehydration and point to the importance of starting our day with some water to replenish our supplies.

As with our nutrition, hydration is a critical part of our self care journey for us to pay attention to the signals our body is giving us and ensure that we are providing it with what it needs.

Key Takeaways

- Being dehydrated can affect our mood as well as our body.

- How we drink is an important aspect of proper hydration.

- Do NOT drink sugar!

- Our body gives us signs when it begins to become mildly dehydrated.

- Drink a glass of water first thing in the morning.

In the next chapter, you will learn...

How our breath can be one of the greatest tools we have to remaining calm and in control during a stressful situation.

Chapter Eight: Breath

We take on average 22,000 breaths per day. Most of those breaths are entirely passive in that we pay little to no attention to them. Even though we are not consciously aware of every breath that we take, our brain is. Every single time we breathe we send a signal to our brain to let it know if we perceive our environment to be safe or threatening, and it triggers a series of physiological and psychological responses as a result.

Imagine you are reading this book right now when suddenly someone starts banging on your front door. The first thing you do in that moment is take a big gasp and hold your breath. This alerts the brain that there is a potentially dangerous situation about to occur, which triggers multiple physiological responses such as an elevated heart rate. After that initial gasp, your breathing then becomes fast and shallow, breathing predominantly from the upper part of the lungs. This triggers the sympathetic nervous system which prepares you for a fight or flight response. You make your way to the door and realise it is your best friend playing a prank on you. You let out a sigh of relief and over a few minutes, your breath begins to return to a normal rate signalling to your brain that the threat has gone, putting you slowly back into a more restful state.

Our breathing changes in this way any time we perceive a situation to be threatening, whether we are being chased by a lion or we have to speak up in a meeting. If we feel afraid of a situation, our breathing will change. This is a really useful survival strategy if we are in a life or death situation. But if we are not, this can cause us to feel even more anxious and afraid and cause a whole host of issues.

When you look at a baby sleeping, you will notice that their belly will move up and down rhythmically. We are all born breathing from our diaphragm muscle which is the large 'parachute type' skeletal muscle which sits below the ribs. When we breathe in this muscle moves to create space in the lower lungs which fill with air. When we breathe out the muscle relaxes and returns to its resting position, to help force the air out of our lungs on an exhale. Breathing this way most of the time has many benefits, but importantly it helps our brain know that in that moment we are safe.

If the baby becomes afraid, it will move to breathing rapidly from the upper lungs but once it feels safe, it will return to breathing from the diaphragm muscle once more.

Unfortunately, as we get older, we begin to learn bad breathing habits and do not always return to deep diaphragmatic breathing. This can be due to extended periods of stress, illness, smoking or vaping to name a few. Many of us then begin to breathe in a way which confirms to our brain and nervous system that we are not safe, even if we are sat watching the television.

Take a moment now as you read, to pay attention to your own breath. Place one hand on your belly and one on your upper chest, if you are breathing from the upper lungs you will notice more movement in the hand on your upper chest, your breathing will be faster and shallower. If you are breathing from your diaphragm muscle, your hand on your belly will move more which will feel deeper, slower and calmer. You may well realise that even sat reading this book, you are breathing shallowly and thus increasing your body's stress levels.

James Nestor, author of the brilliant book "Breath", has gathered decades of research on breathing and how it impacts our health. He makes a strong case for retraining ourselves to be more functional breathers.

It is unsurprising to realise that as soon as we feel life is challenging, our breathing will become faster, shallower and dysfunctional, which will only amplify our feelings of stress and anxiety.

It is therefore one of the most fundamental parts of self care to begin to pay more attention to our own breath and begin to use it to help us to not only deal with difficult times but to lower stress and improve overall wellbeing. Whilst there are many important elements to breathing better and returning to functional breath, there are three simple steps we can all take to begin this process.

Breathe Through Your Nose

James Nestor and many other breathing experts all state the same thing - we must breathe through our noses. Many research studies point to numerous mental and physical health problems appearing or being exacerbated by us becoming a society of mouth breathers.

As a wise person once told me, "We should breathe through our mouths as often as we eat through our noses!".

Our noses are designed for breathing, not our mouths. Our mouths are designed predominantly for eating and talking and are only to be used to breathe in an emergency situation and / or when we are operating at maximum physical capacity. However, it is our noses that are designed for breathing. When we breathe through the nose, we are using the organ specifically designed for efficient breathing. Our noses filtrate the air, ensuring we are better protected from particles in the air which can make us sick. Our noses also ensure a greater and more efficient breath is taken, enabling us to engage the diaphragm muscle and draw air down to the lower lungs, which reassures the brain that we are safe.

When we breathe through our mouths, there is no filtration of the air and whatever we inhale will go into our body. We also send a signal to our brain that we are feeling threatened, which increases stress chemicals such as adrenaline and cortisol. Mouth breathing also causes us to over breathe, the average number of breaths a person takes today is around 15 per minute yet healthy 'resonance' breath is defined as just 5.5 breaths per minute. Finally, mouth breathing makes it very difficult to take a deep breath into the lower lungs, causing us to shallow breathe.

Whenever I talk to people about changing the way they breathe from the mouth to the nose there are usually some people who say they cannot breathe through their nose as it is always blocked.

This is common when we regularly mouth breathe as the nose is not being used frequently and can become congested. Unless you have a physical blockage, such as a polyp or nasal obstruction, a deviated septum or if you are pregnant, you should be able to unblock your nose with this simple exercise:

****

How to Unblock Your Nose Exercise

Take a normal breath in through the nose as best you can.

Exhale through the nose.

Pinch the nose and nod your head back and fore or get up and walk around for a few steps.

Release and return to nasal breathing for 30 seconds.

Repeat up to 5 times.

****

You will notice that your nose feels much clearer, and breathing through your nose becomes easier.

Exhale Longer

As we have already learned, the way we breathe has a huge impact on how our brain interprets our environment and this is largely due to our Autonomic Nervous System.

As we breathe in, we trigger what is known as the sympathetic nervous system which, for these purposes, can be considered as our inner 'accelerator'. The inhale of a breath prepares the brain and body for action. As we exhale, we trigger the parasympathetic nervous system which can be thought of as our inner 'brake'. It slows the body down, hence we will naturally sigh when we feel relaxed or need to relax.

We can use this knowledge to help our breath trigger a feeling of relaxation when we breathe and especially when we feel stressed. There are many breathing exercises to do this and the most simple format is to make your exhale slightly longer than your inhale. You can count this - for example an inhale of a count of four and an exhale for a count of six - but it becomes more relaxing if you feel this naturally rather than count it.

However my favourite way to trigger relaxation is with something called the "Physiological Sigh". Have you ever noticed that when you have become upset and cried, you will often take some big sniffles and then sigh? This is your body's way of naturally trying to calm and relax you, and we can use this technique anytime we feel anxious.

****

The Physiological Sigh Exercise

Breathe in through the nose once.

Without exhaling, take another breath in through the nose.

Release with an extended exhale through the nose.

Repeat 3 times

****

This pattern of breathing has been proven to help reduce stress and is something that we naturally know. You may notice you do a similar pattern after crying or maybe you have watched a dog settling down to sleep and noticed that they do the double inhale with an extended exhale too!

Breathe Gently

When we are stressed and begin to notice our breath, we naturally try to control it, most of us have encouraged someone who is upset to take some deep breaths to help them calm down. However, what is not helpful is that this often involves taking exaggerated deep breaths which can increase our stress levels.

Instead, it is more useful to focus upon breathing gently rather than the volume of air we take in. As Patrick McKeown (author of the Oxygen Advantage and many other books on breath) describes, try to breathe without moving your nostril hairs.

This encourages us to become more mindful of the breath, to slow the breathing down, to take deep breaths and importantly to make those breaths gentle so as not to stress the respiratory system.

****

Breathe Gently Exercise

Mindfully draw in a slow steady breath through the nose with the intention of the air passing through your nose without disturbing your nasal hairs, notice how much longer you can inhale when breathing like this.

Mindfully exhale the breath through the nose in the same manner. Notice how you can exhale for longer than you inhale. Retain control of the breath until all of the air is expelled. Then repeat.

****

Key Takeaways

- Our breath is constantly telling our brain if our environment is safe or threatening.

- Our noses are designed for breathing, not our mouths.

- When we breathe through our mouths, we increase feelings of stress and anxiety.

- When we exhale, we activate the parasympathetic nervous system which helps us to feel relaxed and safe.

- Breathing gently helps us to be more present.

In the next chapter, you will learn...

The importance of giving your mind the benefit of stillness for you to handle challenging situations and why that may be the most important part of your own self care routine.

Chapter Nine: Stillness

We live in a world which appears to encourage us to be busy, to be loud, to be stimulated and to always be 'doing'. But is this really what we need in order for us to care for ourselves?

So many of us are so used to being constantly stimulated that our ability to be still is something we struggle with. Frequently in my therapy room, when I encounter a client who has neglected their self care, they will inform me that they do not have time to care for themselves or they cannot remember the last time they had a moment to themselves. They will often tell me that they cannot stand being quiet and thrive off being busy, but I find this hard to believe.

Yes, we can all thrive from having purpose and meaning in our life (we will cover that in the next chapter) but having purpose should not mean being incapable of taking some time to just be.

94

French philosopher Blaise Pascal famously stated that "All of man's problems stem from his inability to sit alone in a room for any length of time" and I am inclined to agree with him.

When times are challenging, it is natural for us to feel we have to continually take action towards resolving our problems. But frequently, solving a problem is not always within our power and this drive to keep taking action serves only to overwhelm and exhaust us at a time when we need our energy the most.

In order to practise practical self care, it is important we become more comfortable with being in our own company and give ourselves permission to be still. Here are three of my favourite ways in which we can embrace more stillness in our lives.

You are a Human BEING not a Human Doing

If you have ever looked at Mindfulness as a practice you may well have heard "you are a human being, not a human doing". It underpins many of the core practices of mindfulness, to accept that it is okay for us to 'just be' from time to time and in fact recognise that in our being we can heal, grow and thrive.

If you are someone who feels uncomfortable with doing nothing, it is likely that you have become more removed from yourself and more focussed upon others. Whilst it is commendable to care about others, if we consistently do this to our own detriment, we not only neglect our own needs but we risk becoming depleted and being unable to help others as well.

Every now and then it is useful for us to move from doing to being and to recognise that this is an active choice and not entirely passive.

For most of us, doing has now become our default way to behave and we often do things as an automated behaviour without conscious action. A great example of this is how many of us now scroll our mobile phones.

We find that we pick them up and open applications without being consciously aware of doing so and can quickly lose minutes or even hours of our day. A recent fact I heard, to put this into perspective, was that your average TikTok user now scrolls the height of the Eiffel Tower every single day!

When we choose to operate from being, we make a conscious choice to just be in that moment, to refrain from taking any action.

There is a stark difference between how we engage in our lives when we are in 'being mode' and when we are in 'doing mode'.

Being	Doing
Conscious Choice	Automated
Sensing	Analysing
Accepting	Striving
Approach	Avoid
Nourish	Deplete

When we are in doing mode, we are also much more likely to be in our analytical brain, over thinking, over analysing, over focussing and over remembering. This can not only drain us mentally but also develop a pattern of needing to analyse whenever we are not distracted. 'Being' behaviours are more focussed upon using our senses, sitting and listening to the birds, observing the clouds rolling by, feeling our breath move in and out of our body.

Doing behaviours are focussed upon striving to achieve a goal or outcome. We can push ourselves to feel we need to achieve more and berate ourselves when we feel we have not met our target or have failed, whereas being involves accepting the situation as it is.

Accepting a situation as it is, is not giving up or being passive. It is about recognising the things that are out of our control as they are and not wasting energy on wishing they were different. As author and thought leader Eckhart Tolle puts it, "accepting the is-ness of a situation".

When we spend more time being, we are less likely to avoid situations and be trapped in fear. We accept things as they are and therefore do not waste energy trying to change them but save our energy for where our power really lies. When we are constantly in doing mode, we are likely to avoid challenges that we foresee and become stressed about potentially difficult situations that may arise for fear of not being in control.

Finally, when we spend more time being we nourish ourselves, we feel recharged and reconnected to ourselves and others. When we constantly spend our time 'doing' we feel exhausted and depleted with a risk of burning ourselves out and running on empty.

Spending more time 'being' enables us to pay more attention to ourselves, how we feel, to recharge, to nourish ourselves and to accept what is.

Connect to your Heart

The less comfortable we are with stillness, the more stuck in our heads we can be. Most of us know that whenever we are stuck in our heads, we have a tendency to focus more on the negative than the positive. For those overthinkers among us, being stuck in our heads can be the very worst place to be.

We have all been born into a world which values the brain and thinking over any other organ or process. However this has not always been the case. Many ancient cultures and religions considered the heart to be the primary organ and would encourage others to connect with their heart to receive the answers to any questions they may have had.

When your thoughts, emotions, and intentions are in sync, you gain a deep sense of harmony and calm within yourself, as well as a more meaningful connection with everything and everyone around you.

We are often unaware of how powerful our hearts are and that our hearts are constantly sending information to our brain to signal how we are feeling.

Our heart possesses a network of 40,000 neurons called "sensory neurites" which provide a direct line of communication to the brain. These thousands of neurons can sense, process information, make decisions and even demonstrate a type of learning and memory.

Research from The HeartMath Institute illustrates that when we begin to listen to our hearts more, we can create heart / brain coherence which has been shown to have multiple benefits to us including:

- Reducing stress and anxiety by reducing the stress hormone cortisol.

- Improving our immune system.

- Releasing the anti-aging hormone (DHEA).

- Improving our sleep.

- Improving the functioning of the nervous and digestive systems.

- Increasing our concentration.

The most simple way to do this is to spend one to five minutes a day sitting in silence and slowing down your breath, then focus upon a positive emotion, feeling it emanate from the heart such as love, joy or gratitude. However, I love the following exercise which is a combination of the heart coherence exercise and a mindful meditation known as the Meta or Loving Kindness meditation. It is simple and can be done in 5 minutes but you can do it as slowly as you wish.

****

Heart Coherence Exercise

Sit somewhere quiet where you will not be disturbed.

Sit comfortably and focus upon feeling your feet fully connected to the floor.

Close your eyes if you feel comfortable to do so.

Begin to focus upon your breath and start to slow it down, feeling the breath coming in and out of the nose.

As you relax, lift your left hand to sit on your heart.

Feel that physical connection of your heart and your hand to encourage your awareness to move down from your brain and into your heart.

Consider someone you find it easy to love and imagine they are stood in front of you.

As you imagine them there, allow your heart to send those feelings of love to that person.

Silently say as if directed to that person; "May you be happy, may you be healthy, may you be safe, may you live in peace".

Sit with those feelings for a moment.

Now bring to mind someone you feel neutral towards, maybe a neighbour or colleague.

Imagine them in front of you and feel compassion extend from your heart to theirs.

Silently repeat; "May you be happy, may you be healthy, may you be safe, may you live in peace".

Sit with those feelings for a moment.

Now bring to mind someone you find challenging. Do not let your brain think -

just have a sense of this person as a human being in front of you and allow yourself to feel compassion for them.

Silently repeat; "May you be happy, may you be healthy, may you be safe, may you live in peace".

Sit with those feelings for a moment.

Now imagine a mirror is in front of you and you see yourself. Pass no judgement, just have a sense of yourself and allow compassion to be extended to you.

Silently repeat "May I be happy, may I be healthy, may I be safe and may I live in peace".

Sit with those feelings as long as you wish.

Slowly begin to bring your awareness back to the room and allow yourself to become more present in the moment once more.

****

This exercise is a beautiful practice to incorporate into your daily self care routine but is especially powerful if you are dealing with a difficult person and / or are feeling stuck in your head.

Practise Wu Wei

When we feel under pressure from life, whether a health, work or family challenge, we often feel greatest pressure in the expectation of us needing to take action right now. This can cause us additional stress and often for us to make the wrong decision, as we do not make the best decisions when we are stressed.

There is a fantastic Taoist philosophy which I find incredibly useful during these times. It is known as the practice of "Wu Wei" which roughly means "The action of inaction".

During times when we do not know what to do, it is very often the right thing to do nothing and this is where Wu Wei can be applied. It is not passive, nor is it about opting out of making a decision; it is making a very definite decision to do nothing in this very moment.

Embracing the philosophy of Wu Wei can help us to be more still and accepting of a situation without the tendency of making a knee jerk reaction which could potentially worsen the situation.

The next time you feel you do not know what to do and have the luxury of some time, take it as an opportunity of practising Wu Wei and you are likely to find that, very often, things work out when we do not jump in and try to control or fix them immediately. At the very least, you will give yourself time to allow your stress to calm and be in a better frame of mind to make a decision with more rational thought.

Key Takeaways

- We have been conditioned to believe we should always be doing something but there is a lot of benefit in learning to be still.

- It is useful to remember we are human beings, not human doings.

- When we focus upon being, we allow ourselves to be more present and do what is right for us.

- It can be useful to focus less on our brain at times and allow ourselves to move down into our hearts.

- Sometimes the action of inaction, Wu Wei, is entirely the right thing for us to choose to do.

In the next chapter, you will learn...

Why living with purpose could be the key to finding meaning, connection, gratitude and joy within our lives.

Chapter Ten: Purpose

There are many people who go through their lives with a deep sense of knowing their own purpose. They seem to know why they are here, where their strengths lie and know what they offer to the World. However, arguably many more people have a sense of knowing they must have a purpose but can spend their entire lives not knowing what it is nor how to find it.

This leaves so many of us feeling lost and unfulfilled in many aspects of our lives. When life becomes challenging, it is even more pivotal for us to have a sense of purpose or else we find ourselves floundering in the absurdity of why we are being challenged so much.

Palliative care nurse, Bronnie Ware, spent many years sitting with people as they reached the end of their lives and began to make notes of their thoughts as they came to the end. She noticed recurring themes of regrets her patients would share with her as they faced their own mortality and wrote a blog on the subject which eventually became a best selling book "The Top Five Regrets of The Dying". The top 5 regrets of the dying as Ware experienced are:

1. I wish I'd had the courage to live a life true to myself, not the life others expected of me.

2. I wish I didn't work so hard.

3. I wish I'd had the courage to express my feelings.

4. I wish I had stayed in touch with my friends.

5. I wish I had let myself be happier.

Four out of five of these top 5 regrets all relate to living our truth and fulfilling our purpose in life. Whether we end up in a career chosen by pushy parents, or falling into a job because it offered a decent salary or prospects, many of us end up trapping ourselves into living without passion or sense of purpose and it seems many of us will regret that at the end of our lives.

When we begin to consider having a purpose, many of us envisage something that must be grand, impactful and world changing such as saving a rare animal from extinction or rebuilding a village that has experienced a natural disaster. Of course, there are indeed people who make tasks like these their great mission but if we consider all of us to be here to carry out such grand purposes, then most of us will inevitably be unfulfilled.

It is my experience from working with people to help them find purpose and meaning that our sense of purpose does not need to be something that changes the world, only something that changes 'our world'. It appears to me, that in order for us to find purpose and meaning in our every day life then we need to tick at least one of these boxes:

1. Impacting and helping other people.

2. Impacting and helping the planet.

3. Impacting and helping animals.

I cannot think of anyone who has a sense of purpose who does not in some way feel fulfilment from making a difference in at least one of these areas.

Having a sense of purpose is crucial to our own self care, self confidence and growth as without it, we risk living someone else's purpose and / or feeling a sense of pointlessness.

Your purpose gives you a reason to follow through and do whatever it takes to create the outcome you desire. Whereas an outcome (or result) produces focus, a purpose gives you drive. For example, it's one thing to say, "I want to become a millionaire." It's another thing to say, "I want to become a millionaire because I will be able to help my children; make a difference in the world; develop the pride of knowing that I've overcome so many challenges; support the homeless; and create many magical, fun moments for myself and those I love!"

When you fully feel why you are doing something, you will create the emotional excitement, resilience and energy that will give you the drive and momentum to create a positive result.

Therefore, to find your purpose, it is useful to begin by identifying the emotions that you want to experience first. It is in identifying these emotions that you will be able to find your passion and purpose in everything you do!

Childhood Dreams

I believe that as children, we know what we are passionate about and where we find purpose but at that point we do not have the verbal or emotional intelligence to be able to communicate this. So we begin to show it through our imaginative games and often through what we say we want to be or do when we 'grow up'.

As we grow, we become heavily influenced by parents, teachers, friends and the media. As a result we lose this sense of clear purpose and begin living up to the expectations of teachers, parents and society.

I believe that those first dreams we had as a child are the key to us tuning back in to where we can find our purpose. No child ever says they want to be a police officer for the pension nor a doctor for the salary. They are likely to say they want to do these jobs because of the emotions they associate with it, such as helping others. Try the following exercise.

****

Childhood Dreams Exercise

Sit quietly somewhere and ensure you have a pen and paper to hand for this exercise.

Take a moment to close your eyes and draw in a deep breath through the nose and exhale slowly.

Allow yourself to relax and wind down.

In this calm relaxed state, begin to imagine your younger self as far back as you can imagine, see or sense yourself as a small child.

Remember that young child as clearly as you can and then try to remember what the younger version of you enjoyed doing.

Now consider what did you want to be when you grew up? No matter how wacky or silly it may seem, be honest with yourself.

Now move the clock forward a little, imagine yourself as slightly older, maybe a teenager. Had your wishes changed? **Can you remember what you wanted to be at this age?**

Now how about when you left school or university, **what did you want to be then?**

Finally, allow your imagination to wander and ask yourself, **what would you like to do right now** if money, time, age, education were no obstacle?

Do not rush these questions, give yourself time to allow your mind to wander and know that whatever comes up is okay.

When finished, bring yourself back to the room and write down all of your answers.

You may want to repeat this exercise a few times to get fuller answers.

As you look at your responses, begin to consider what emotions you would have thought each 'profession' would have brought you. This is the key to you connecting with what your childhood dreams were pushing you towards.

Write out emotions for each age and see if there are recurring themes. These emotions are the ones that light you up and guide you towards your purpose.

****

Follow the Joy

Neuroscientist David Eagleman in his brilliant book "Sum" states that an average person experiences 14 minutes of pure joy in their entire lifetime. When I learned this, it shocked and saddened me that we experience so little joy. Of course, we can experience happiness, thrill and excitement but they do not necessarily equate to joy.

Joy is an emotion reserved largely for those experiences in our life that we consider to be 'exceptional'; the birth of a child, a wedding day, a much anticipated holiday.

However, if we are only to experience joy on those rare occasions, we risk falling into Eagleman's statistic of experiencing only 14 minutes of joy in our lifetime. It is my belief that we can experience far more joy than this but we need to begin by prioritising joy in our lives, which is naturally challenging when we feel under pressure.

Joy is subjective and therefore we can seek to experience it in the every day if we train our brains to do so. Miroslav Volf, Professor of Systematic Theology at Yale Divinity School, states that joy, "is tied to how I perceive things rather than to what things are in themselves". Which means that we can begin to view the world with our 'joy glasses' on a little more, this will help us to see not only beauty in the every day but to also find purpose within that simple act.

One of the most powerful ways I know of training the brain to experience more joy is by teaching the brain to appreciate what we already have. The best way to do this is through practising gratitude. Gratitude is studied under the heading of Positive Psychology and has been described as the most powerful emotion we possess. There are numerous research studies highlighting the benefits of practising gratitude such as feeling happier, visiting the doctor less, improving relationships and much more. The world's leading expert on gratitude is Robert Emmons PhD, and through his research he has found that when people practise gratitude they:

- Have stronger immune systems.
- Are less bothered by aches and pains.
- Have lower blood pressure.
- Exercise more and take better care of their health.
- Sleep longer and feel more refreshed upon waking.
- Have higher levels of positive emotions.
- Are more optimistic and happier.
- Are more helpful, generous, and compassionate.
- Feel less lonely and isolated.
- Are more joyful!

Each of these can lead to us feeling that we have more purpose, passion, joy and connection within our lives and the wonderful aspect of practising gratitude is that there are no negative side effects of doing so.

****

Practising Gratitude Exercise

There are numerous ways to practise gratitude, from a simple journal detailing 3 things you are grateful for every day to writing letters of thanks to someone.

In order for you to receive the maximum benefits of gratitude, try this exercise.

Sit quietly with some paper and a pen.

Begin to think of some people whom you are grateful for and write down their names and importantly, why you are grateful for them.

Now think of some experiences you are grateful for and again write them down with some detail.

Now consider material items you are grateful for and again write them down and explain why.

Finally, write down some aspects of yourself you are grateful for.

Take your time through this exercise and give yourself plenty of time to reflect on your answers.

Repeat regularly.

****

Make a Pledge

Choosing to live with more purpose can highlight areas in your life which are lacking or do not fulfil you, which can be confronting. The aim is not to completely redesign your life overnight, but to start to encourage you to see more purpose, passion and joy in the life you currently have even if you know over time that things will need to change.

When life feels challenging and daunting, it can be easy to let this aspect of our self care to really slip by us and not be prioritised. But I also know that when we do that, we feel more demotivated and lost than before.

A simple way to begin to deal with finding more purpose in your life is to begin to reconnect with the things that make your soul sing. Can you remember what they are? It is okay if you do not.

Years ago, I found myself entirely lost and disconnected from who I really was. I had spent the majority of my adult life trying to please everyone else and be what I thought they wanted me to be. It was not until I made some big changes that I realised I did not even know what I liked anymore, from food to music! I was lost.

This was daunting and upsetting. I had buried who I was under layers of protection, and rediscovering 'me' felt like an impossible task. Instead of seeing that I needed to work that out in one go, I did something a little kinder for myself. I decided to make a pledge to myself that went as follows:

"I promise to do one thing every day that is just for myself, even if only for five minutes"

This felt do-able and did not overwhelm me. Little did I know how powerful it would prove to be. Making this pledge meant that, even if only for five minutes, I gave myself permission to care for myself, to connect with myself and to follow something that brought me joy. This ranged from a quiet cup of tea to a day out with my best friend to signing up to a course. Over a period of months, I started to recognise what I did and did not enjoy, I connected with what gave me purpose and I started to break away from the masks that I had worn for years.

If you are lost right now, make this pledge to yourself, and ensure that you stick to it.

Key Takeaways

- Our purpose does not have to be something that is world changing.

- Some of the biggest regrets people have in their lives connect to not living their purpose.

- Our childhood dreams can reveal emotions we sought out when we were younger which may still be relevant to us today.

- Joy can be cultivated by living with more gratitude.

- Gratitude has significant benefits to our life.

- By making a pledge to prioritise ourselves, even if only for five minutes a day, we give ourselves permission to be our authentic selves.

In the next chapter, you will learn...

Why our relationships are a crucial aspect not only to our application of self care but within every area of our wellbeing.

Chapter Eleven: Relationships

No matter how antisocial we may believe we are, human beings are highly social animals. It is difficult for a human being to survive in isolation and nigh on impossible for one to thrive in isolation.

Whenever I train on resilience, I always ask delegates what resources they rely upon when they go through a difficult time and in all my years of doing this, the top answer has always been the same - "other people".

No matter how much we enjoy our own company, we intuitively know that if we are going through a challenging time then we are better positioned to survive it if we have other people around us. In primitive times, that would have looked like us calling our tribe members to scare off a predator. In our modern times that can look like telling a friend about your difficult day, asking a colleague for help or seeking out therapy to deal with a challenging problem. We are hardwired for social connection, especially when we are struggling.

On top of our need for social support at difficult times, there are countless research studies out there which highlight the correlation between the quality of our relationships and the quality of our life. Satisfying relationships with others not only make us happier but have been shown to make us healthier and even live longer.

Despite us living in a world where we are now more connected than ever with the World seeming smaller and smaller, the number of people experiencing loneliness and isolation is at an all time high. We now have a larger number of 'friends' or 'followers' but we feel less connected.

Our relationships are a core need for our wellbeing and in some ways can be considered in the same way as our need for food. We can have lots of food around us and eat all day long but if it does not give us the nutrition we need, we can still be unhealthy and unsatisfied. Relationships can be a lot like that; we can be surrounded by hundreds of people and still feel that we are lonely and not receiving the nourishment we need.

One thing that seems evident with relationships is that it is not a numbers game. It is far more likely down to how connected we feel, and when our relationships satisfy us, we benefit in ways we may not expect.

This is highlighted wonderfully in a study originally carried out in 1938 when scientists began tracking the health of 268 Harvard sophomores during the Great Depression. The study was intended to reveal clues as to how to lead happy and healthy lives.

This study became one of the world's longest longitudinal studies and expanded to include the children the men had. Over the years, researchers studied the participants' health trajectories and their broader lives, including their triumphs and failures in careers and marriage, and the findings have produced startling lessons.

"The surprising finding is that our relationships and how happy we are in our relationships has a powerful influence on our health," said Robert Waldinger, director of the study, a psychiatrist at Massachusetts General Hospital and a professor of psychiatry

at Harvard Medical School. "Taking care of
your body is important, but tending to your
relationships is a form of self-care too. That, I
think, is the revelation".

Loneliness is Bad for Your Health

One hundred years ago our ancestors
would have been immersed in their
communities and living with extended families,
they would have had social contact and
support every single day. Yet today, some
people can go days, weeks or even months
without social connection and we know that
has a detrimental effect on our wellbeing.

As we have already seen, studies have
consistently shown that positive social
connections are good for our health and poor
or no relationships are bad for our health.
According to Julianne Holt-Lunstad, a
psychology professor at Brigham Young
University, insufficient social connection is a
bigger risk factor to our health than obesity and
the equivalent of smoking up to 15 cigarettes a
day.

It's been well established that lonely people are more likely than the nonlonely to die from cardiovascular disease, cancer, respiratory illness, and gastrointestinal causes. One study found that those with fewer than three people they could confide in and count on for social support were more than twice as likely to die from heart disease than those with more confidants. They were also roughly twice as likely to die of all causes, even when age, income, and smoking status were comparable.

The problem with loneliness however is that even though it is a core human need to have social connection, when we feel lonely we do not always seek to satisfy our need.

If we consider feeling hunger, the pangs of hunger begin gently at first and we can ignore them but eventually they become more and more painful until we have to seek out some food in order to relieve the pain.

Loneliness works in a very similar way, with the pangs of loneliness being gentler at first and gradually increasing. However, unlike with hunger, the more loneliness grows, the less likely we are to seek out the very thing that will remove the pain and the more likely we are to isolate ourselves further.

When we feel lonely, it is important to recognise that this feeling is there in order for you to satisfy your lack and not to cause you suffering. It is then useful to see loneliness as a need which needs fulfilling.

1. Acknowledge that you feel lonely.

2. Focus on how you can help someone else.

3. Focus upon what you are grateful for.

4. Initiate dialogue with family, friends, or associates. Ideally in person.

5. Learn something new. This can boost self-confidence and provide new opportunities to connect with others.

6. Consider a counsellor or therapist. You may need support

in working through the factors that contribute to your feeling lonely.

Be Honest

Developing good relationships requires trust. We are often aware of needing to trust others but do not always consider that we need to be trustworthy too. A way in which we can improve the quality of our relationships is by being more honest in the ones that matter.

Many of us put on a front or wear a mask even with the people closest to us for fear of judgment and / or rejection. However, this is draining and prevents us from having healthy relationships.

Of course, we do not need to tell anyone and everyone exactly how we feel but if we hide our truth from those closest to us there will always be a barrier preventing the relationship from creating any depth.

A great example of where we are often dishonest is in our response to a really simple question. When a friend or family asks you

"How are you?", how do you reply? With people you do not feel close to, it is likely you will have a 'stock response' where you say a reply which you do not even think about, something like "fine" or "Not bad". However, how do you respond to this question with the people closest to you? This is when it really matters.

If we hide how we really are, we stop ourselves from connecting. When you are next asked this question by someone you trust, I challenge you to give a more honest response and when you ask someone this question, I challenge you to really hear what they tell you.

The 5 People

Having good social support is critical for self care but we also need to be aware that we can have different people in our lives to depend upon in different scenarios and not everyone around us makes us feel good.

Your best friend may be an amazing person to chat to when you are having relationship problems, but maybe they do not understand your work and so when a work problem arises, you may need to talk to a colleague or mentor. We can often make situations more challenging by seeking out the help of the wrong person at a difficult time. Some people, with the best intentions, may cause you to worry more or feel more anxious in a situation than you were in the first place.

Motivational Speaker Jim Rohn famously said "You become the average of the five people you spend most of your time with". This was based upon something called "The 5 Chimps Theory" established from findings in zoology which shows that when a new chimp is introduced to an existing troop of chimps, it will mimic and copy the behaviours of the existing troop in order to be fully accepted.

Human beings, by Jim Rohn's example, are very similar in that we will also mimic behaviours, values and beliefs of those we engage with the most to become accepted, until we become the 'average' of the five people we spend most of our time with.

Take a moment now to jot down the names of the five people you engage with most frequently, you will notice that this may not necessarily be a list of the five people you love the most as you are likely to engage with work colleagues or house mates more than some family or friends.

The 5 People I spend most of my time with	Nourish	Deplete

Once you have written down their names, spend a moment asking yourself "When I spend time with this person, how do they make me feel? Do they nourish or deplete me?".

Everyone and everything we engage with has the ability to both nourish – make us feel good, recharged, energised or deplete – make us feel drained, negative and tired.

Of course, from time to time we can all oscillate between being nourishing and depleting but consider the average of your time spent with that person. Are they generally more nourishing or depleting?

As you look at your list, you may notice you have more 'depleters' than 'nourishers' which will inevitably leave you feeling depleted once you spend time with them. You may realise that some of these people are not good for you and decide to create some more distance from them. However some of these people may be unavoidable, such as a colleague or a loved one.

If this is the case, then you do not need to cut them out of your life, but simply become aware of how they make you feel. Knowing that when you are feeling down these are probably not the people to turn to. I also suggest that you make a plan for when you spend time with them, knowing that they can be depleting can help you plan something nourishing to do after engaging with them.

Be mindful of how people make you feel, choose nourishers wherever you can and know that you do not need to share everything with everyone.

Key Takeaways

- Our relationships have a huge impact on our health and happiness.

- Fostering positive relationships is seen as an important part of self care.

- Loneliness is a sign that we are lacking the social connection we need.

- To deepen our closest relationships, it is important that we are honest with ourselves and others.

- We become the average of the five people we spend most of our time with.

- People can nourish and deplete us.

- We can have good relationships with people but do not necessarily need to tell them everything nor ask for their advice in every situation.

In the next chapter, you will learn...

How to create new behaviours to implement self care practices into your every day life.

Part III: Putting Things into Action

Chapter Twelve: Creating New Behaviours

We have covered eight key aspects of self care with multiple examples and ideas of how we could improve each area. However most of us recognise that change can be hard! It would therefore be understandable if right now you were thinking "I need to change so much, I don't know where to start".

Human beings are creatures of habit. We like to do what we have always done, even if we know that is not helpful or even harmful to us. Even when we recognise that a change in behaviour could yield us countless positive benefits, we can still find the change difficult and end up self sabotaging.

I have met so many clients who get frustrated with this behaviour and feel as if there must be something wrong with them as they believe other people do not do this. They do!

136

Our brain's primary purpose above everything else is to keep us safe. That is it! Your brain does not care if you are happy, in love, calm - it cares that you are alive. It does this in countless ways every moment of the day, but in terms of our behaviour, it does this by assuming if we are alive today, then what we did yesterday generally worked for us. Even if what we did yesterday was feel anxious, overwhelmed, self critical, your brain will still see it as a success as you survived.

Therefore, when we come to identify harmful behaviours that we may have, we tend to notice resistance in our brain being willing to give up the unhelpful behaviour.

Knowing and accepting that this occurs is a useful first step. It is also useful to know that, according to a Duke University study, we spend around 40% of our waking day on 'autopilot', doing things that we have done every other day without any particular conscious involvement. This can be really helpful - every morning you do not need to feel confused as you begin to contemplate brushing your teeth. You have done this so many times that you simply grab the toothbrush, squeeze on some toothpaste and begin brushing, probably whilst your brain is contemplating something completely unrelated. Sometimes, we do things on such autopilot that we even forget if we have done it – did you brush your teeth today? This kind of behaviour helps us to conserve brain energy and enables us to perform repeated tasks with little interruption. However, we also perform autopilot tasks on lots of our behaviours which may not be as helpful.

A great example of our autopilot behaviour is how frequently we reach for our phones (there are many studies on this with varying figures but an average figure is once every 4 minutes!). Consider your phone usage. Do you find yourself scrolling when the TV adverts come on, when someone leaves a room, when you are sat waiting for someone? Most of us do this entirely on autopilot.

Changing our behaviours therefore can be challenging for everyone but there are little tools we can use to help our new desired behaviours become our new autopilot behaviours.

1. Start Small

Every single habit and behaviour expert all appear to agree that in order for us to make a long term change in our behaviours, the smaller we start the better. BJ Fogg (author of Tiny Habits) talks about wanting to floss his teeth and how many times he failed at this new behaviour, until he decided to challenge himself to floss just one tooth. So small, it was unlikely to make a difference to his gum health but also so small, it was harder for his brain to object to the behaviour. As flossing one tooth became easier, some days he would do more and eventually, over time, he was able to gradually increase that habit to more and more teeth until he was used to doing the whole mouth.

2. Make it Easy

When creating a new behaviour, make it as easy as possible to carry it through. If you say you want to drink more water but never carry a drink around with you, you are unlikely to do it. If you want to go the gym more but your gym is miles and miles away, it is likely to fail.

Consider your new behaviour and make it as easy as possible to do it.

3. Be Consistent

You are a human being and therefore are likely to fail from time to time. However many of us sabotage ourselves once we feel we have failed at our new behaviour. Maybe you commit to not eating processed food and then on a tiring day, you submit to having a pizza. We can often feel that once we have broken our new behaviour then there is no point in continuing, but research shows no measurable impact on missing your behaviour once. What you do not want to do is do that more than once in a row. That's when a slip up becomes your new behaviour.

Identify Your Kryptonite

As you have read this book, you have probably recognised that there are areas in your life that you want to improve. However I encourage you to first think about what is the one behaviour that you are currently doing which is having the most negative impact on your wellbeing – one thing that if you managed to stop doing right now, you know your overall wellbeing would improve. It may be one of the following, or you may have your own:

I drink too much alcohol.

I am going to bed way too late.

I am eating too much junk food.

I am hanging around with the wrong people.

I use my phone too much.

I don't move enough.

I am too busy.

When you identify the one behaviour you need to stop doing, consider that to be your very own kryptonite. You probably know that Superman only had one weakness, which was kryptonite, and we are using that same concept.

As you have identified your kryptonite, make a pledge that from today, you will stop doing this one thing.

Identify Your Keystone

A keystone is the centre stone used in an archway. It is the pivotal piece of an arch and without it, the rest of the arch would collapse.

As with your kryptonite, now consider what is the one thing you could do right now that would improve your wellbeing. I would suggest thinking about each of the eight areas we have covered and choosing one which you know will have a positive knock on effect to the others. For example:

My keystone behaviour is sleep, when I get enough sleep it is easier for me to support my other healthy choices throughout the day.

My keystone behaviour is movement, when I have moved my body I am energised and find challenges easier to face.

My keystone behaviour is purpose, when I remind myself of my purpose then I know what I am doing and feel driven to achieve my goals.

As you identify your keystone behaviour, focus upon this one as your starting point to improving your self care.

Key Takeaways

- Creating new behaviours can be difficult as the brain wants to keep us safe.

- To change behaviour, it is best to begin small.

- Identifying your kryptonite, the one behaviour that is negatively impacting your wellbeing, is a useful place to begin.

- Identifying your keystone will help begin the process of practising daily self care.

In the next chapter, we will …

Reflect on everything we have learned throughout the book.

Conclusion

Self care is a fundamental aspect to our overall health and wellbeing and yet many of us can neglect even our most basic of needs. This becomes especially difficult whenever we face a challenging period in our life. Whilst there are many acts of self care, everything we do for ourselves could be considered an act of self care if it is nourishing. We have specifically looked at the eight basics of self care:

- Sleep
- Movement
- Nutrition
- Hydration
- Breath
- Stillness
- Purpose
- Relationships

As we have explored the concept of self care, we have identified not only how crucial it is, but also how common it is for many of us to have barriers to caring for ourselves. This book is designed to encourage you to overcome those barriers and recognise that you are worthy of care and attention. In fact when you give these things to yourself you also show others that they are worthy of the same.

If you have a challenging relationship with yourself right now and find it hard to like yourself, please know that tiny acts of self care can improve this relationship.

Consider this, I ask an arachnophobe if they will care for my tarantula* Mavis. I tell them that Mavis needs cuddles, hand feeding and to be told how beautiful she is every day. How easy do you think it would be for the arachnophobe to do this? It would be nigh on impossible! Because it is impossible to care for something you hate.

Now relate this back to yourself. If you are being mean to yourself and have never found it easy to show kindness and compassion to yourself, you may have a similar aversion to my example. But tiny steps towards self kindness are the key to realising that, just like Mavis, you are lovable, worthy, and deserving.

(*I do not have a pet tarantula named Mavis)

Further Help & Support

If you are struggling right now, please know that there is a great deal of help and support available to you. You can of course reach out to your GP who will be able to help and / or advise you of local resources available. You could also reach out to a counsellor or therapist.

There are also countless websites that can help and support you too. Some general ones I feel offer great resources are:

MIND – www.mind.org.uk

Samaritans – www.samaritans.org

Campaign Against Living Miserably (CALM) - https://www.thecalmzone.net/

Resources & Recommended Reading

ROBBINS, Tony - Why do people do what they do? | 6 human needs (tonyrobbins.com)

MILLER, et al (2019) Examining the self-care practices of child welfare workers: A national perspective

RIEGEL, et al (2017) Self-Care for the Prevention and Management of Cardiovascular Disease and Stroke | Journal of the American Heart Association (ahajournals.org)

WALKER, M (2017) Why We Sleep. The New Science of Sleep and Dreams.

WAGNER, FOLK et al (2019) Recreational Screen Time Behaviors during the COVID-19 Pandemic in the U.S.

MEADOWS, GUY Dr (2014) The Sleep Book. How to Sleep Well Every Night.

MEDINA, John (2009) Brain Rules. 12 Principles for Surviving and Thriving at Work, Home and School.

MANDASGER, HARB, CREMER et al (2018) Association of Cardiorespiratory Fitness With Long-term Mortality Among Adults Undergoing

Exercise Treadmill Testing | Cardiology | JAMA Network Open | JAMA Network

McGONIGAL, Kelly (2019) The Joy of Movement: How Exercise Helps Us Find Happiness, Hope, Connection, and Courage

NEFFENDORF, Sam (2022) Home - Sam Neffendorf (eftnow.co.uk)

MASENTO et al (2014) Effects of hydration status on cognitive performance and mood | British Journal of Nutrition | Cambridge Core

BLOSSOM, Scott (2023) Doctor Blossom

HYMAN, Mark (2021) Food Fix: How to Save Our Health, Our Economy, Our Communities and Our Planet – One Bite at a Time

NESTOR, James (2021) Breath: The New Science of a Lost Art

McKEOWN, Patrick (2020) The Oxygen Advantage

HEARTMATH, Institute HeartMath Institute

EAGLEMAN, David (2009) Sum: Forty Tales From After Lives

EMMONS, Robert (2008) Thanks! How Practicing Gratitude Can Make You Happier

WALDINGER, Robert (2023) The Good Life. Lessons From The World's Longest Study on Happiness

WARE, Bronnie (2012) The Top Five Regrets of the Dying: A Life Transformed by the Dearly Departing

HOLT-LUNSTAD, Julianne et al (2010) Social Relationships and Mortality Risk: A Meta-analytic Review

FOGG, BJ (2020) Tiny Habits. Why Starting Small Makes Lasting Changes Easy

Acknowledgments

For more than a decade, I have been working with companies, groups and individuals to help them improve their overall health, wellbeing and happiness. During that time, it has become so evident to me that much of our own suffering and struggles comes from our not being prepared to prioritise ourselves. This book is the product of the people whom I have met who over time have been open to believing that they are worthy of caring for themselves and for each of those I am grateful.

Extra special thanks to my great friend Gemma, who not only supports me constantly but has also taken the time to proof read my work, it is so appreciated!

I am also grateful for those people in my life who have shown me that I am worthy of self care too, especially my darling husband Tom. When we first met, I was lost, in pain and believed I was worthless. One fateful lunch with him changed my life. During that lunch he asked me what my dreams were. I paused for a long time and felt tears prick my eyes. I realised in that moment that I had become so focussed upon pleasing everyone else, I had totally neglected myself to the point that I no longer even dared dream of something better.

Tom showed me I was worthy and to this day encourages me to chase my dreams and be selfish whenever I need to. I am forever in awe of him and grateful for him.

Finally, I am grateful to my parents, Lynda & Tom. My mum Lynda is someone who epitomises being a mum. She states that it is all she ever really wanted and to this day dedicates herself to her family. However I have noticed over the years that she too has learned that you have to be kinder to yourself and do things for yourself too.

My Dad Tom will forever be my hero. Unfortunately, my dad died suddenly and unexpectedly in 2019, a day that forever changed my life and changed me as a person. My Dad was unapologetically himself, he never did things to please or impress others but lived a life with love for all those he cared about. He taught me that being myself was enough. I am who I am because I am his daughter.

Finally, none of my work would be possible without the people who ask for the content I create so a huge thank you to everyone who engages on social media, sends emails and purchases my books. I sincerely hope it guides you to being kinder to yourself every day.

About the Author

Lianne Weaver is an author, speaker, trainer and therapeutic coach with more than a decade of experience working within wellbeing and personal development.

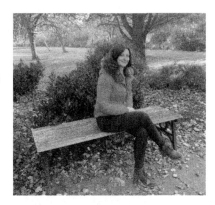

After gaining a BA (Hons) Education whilst specialising in psychology, Lianne dreamed of becoming a play therapist. Despite completing the course to do so, her personal circumstances meant she needed to find employment quickly after qualifying and so she began work within a call centre at a financial institution. Quickly, she was promoted into Human Resources where she was then sponsored to do a Post Grad in Human Resource Management which she really enjoyed.

However, shortly after qualifying, she discovered she was pregnant and knew she would need to put her career aside to care for her daughter. As time went by, returning to a career in HR seemed more and more unlikely and after several diversions, Lianne decided to retrain as a Bookkeeper. She did so and began preparing a small bookkeeping practice from home whilst she continued studying as an Accounting Technician (AAT).

As her daughter began school, Lianne set up a bookkeeping and accountancy practice which created an illusion of success all around her. However, internally, Lianne felt unhappy, lost and afraid. She had realised she was in a life she did not like nor was healthy for her and yet felt unable to make any changes.

Eventually, in 2010, Lianne essentially left her life with her daughter, her dog and very little money. In essence she had to start her life all over again and struggled with this until she decided to venture into studying holistic therapies. She took courses on Reiki, Aromatherapy, Massage and more and started a small holistic therapy practice. Here, she met many interesting people and was invited to speak at an organisation who subsequently asked if she could deliver a training programme on wellbeing.

Since that time, Lianne has created over 100 courses on topics ranging from stress to forgiveness to meditation and much more, most of which are CPD accredited. She has continued to learn and moved into talking therapies such as Emotional Freedom Technique (EFT), Neuro-Linguistic Programming (NLP), Coaching and Havening. Her business, Beam Development & Training Ltd, now delivers wellbeing and personal development training in organisations around the world and she still enjoys working with clients on a one to one basis as a Therapeutic Coach when she is able.

Lianne has worked as a wellbeing and personal development expert for large organisations, been on many international podcasts and has spoken on stages as a leader in her field.

Lianne lives with her husband Tom and dog Dave and enjoys nothing more than being with her family, especially her daughter.

Online Content

For further resources including worksheets and videos please visit https://www.beamtraining.co.uk/beamresource s or scan the QR code below.

Printed in Great Britain
by Amazon

33005448R00096